Table of Contents

INTRODUCTION

Unfortunately, liver disease in dogs is a common occurrence. Your veterinarian will help you develop an evidence-based plan to alleviate the symptoms, which will likely involve tests, medication and diet. This BOOK will discuss specifically the dietary changes you can make for your dog with liver disease and to prevent the ones that don't have from having.

Canine Liver Disease (CLD) is rather common in dogs. Some breeds are more susceptible to it than others. However, the symptoms and effects of the disease are the same for every dog. CLD is a big problem since it compromises the functioning of your dog's liver. This disease can become serious. However, it can also be brought under control and even cured. One of the best ways of dealing with CLD is diet control. Today, we're going to talk about homemade dog food for liver disease patients. In this article, we shall identify food items that are beneficial for a dog's liver and how they can be used to fight CLD. Before we get into curing and managing CLD, let's develop an understanding of the disease itself.

CHAPTER ONE

What is a Liver Disease in Dogs?

Liver is an important organ in a dog's body that acts as a cleaning system, removing toxins and waste, and producing bile for better digestion. When dog's liver gets compromised, the build-up of toxins and waste can affect other organs and cause further dangerous health issues.

Causes of liver disease in dogs may be injuries, poor diet, aging or genes. It can also be a result of some infection or trauma in that area, as well as other diseases affecting the liver or even medications. Some breeds, like Doberman Pinschers and West Highland Terriers, are at higher risk of liver disease according to studies.

If you suspect that your dog is suffering from a liver disease, take him to your vet immediately. Early detection can help in treating the problem and, thanks to liver's ability to regenerate itself, it can also lead to complete recovery, with the right treatment using medication and proper diet for dogs with liver disease.

Diet for Dogs With Liver Disease

Since the causes of the liver disease vary, the ways to deal with this problem can also be different. Developing a plan with your vet is crucial based on the causes of liver disease, but dietary changes can certainly help your dog.

Dietary Guidelines

Some people choose to feed their dogs raw diets. Even though raw feeding is still a highly debatable topic, it's clear that practicing safe raw feeding principles can be healthier and easier for the dog's liver than many commercial dog food brands, particularly the cheap non-prescription formulas.

There are many benefits when it comes to homemade meals. The major ones being; fresh, quality ingredients, no additives and chemicals, and complete control over what goes into your dog's belly. Dogs with liver disease needs to be fed meals that:

Reduce stress on their liver and provide nutrition that boosts liver regeneration.

Provide the dog with balanced nutrition to maintain their health.

Prevent the buildup of harmful substances in the body by using selective ingredients.

Use food items that help minimize the effects of toxins already present in the body.

Now, a dog with liver disease will have a limited diet. There's a list of food items that fall off the menu since they promote toxin build up. One common misconception about CLD is that dogs cannot be fed protein if their liver is unwell. This misconception stems from the fact that some protein sources encourage the buildup of ammonia in the body. Ammonia can be quite harmful if its buildup is left unchecked. However, having CLD doesn't mean that your dog shouldn't have protein. In fact, protein is an essential nutrient that your dog needs to heal faster. Instead of prohibiting protein from their diet, you should go for protein sources that produce lesser ammonia. Keep in mind that while protein shouldn't be banned, its quantity should be reduced.

You also need to reduce the amount of fat that your dog eats. The liver plays an important role in the body's ability to breakdown fat. You want to reduce the amount of fat in your dog's diet and also cut back on protein. Make sure that what protein you do give to your dog comes from quality, easy to digest sources. Ideally, you want quality proteins that are combined with essential amino acids as well. Lastly, you want to increase the amount of fiber that your dog eats. Fiber helps the digestive system. Also, most sources of fiber are rich in nutrients that boost your dog's health as well.

It goes without saying that any pre-packaged dog food cannot meet such selective dietary requirements. This is why homemade food is the best option. Now, before we finally start going through some homemade dog food recipes, let's take a look at some food items that you'd want to include in your dog's diet.

Sources of Fiber And Carbs

Whole Wheat Grain (in bread form)

Oatmeal

Pumpkin

Grounded vegetable skins

Barley

Sources of Quality Proteins

Fish

Lean chicken meat (with the skin)

Eggs

Yogurt (low fat)

Cottage cheese (low fat)

Sources of Fat

Omega 3 fatty acids. Can be found in salmon oil and fish oil (cod liver oil shouldn't be used)

Fat from animal meats (in moderate quantities)

Red meats shouldn't be fed to dogs with liver disease since they produce a higher amount of ammonia.

Important Nutrients

Some nutrients are more important than others for dogs with liver disease, and you should keep that in mind when you plan a diet for your canine.

Protein

The optimal protein intake will vary depending on the stage and type of liver disease. Some types of liver disease will demand protein increase, while other types or stages might require limiting protein. However, for the health of the liver it is important that you feed your dog high-quality protein. In fact, it is a general recommendation to ensure the protein you give to your dog is high quality, but also to feed him in moderate amounts.

The best proteins for increased protein intake are from animal sources. They have the optimal amounts of amino acids which are good for your dog in general, especially for his digestion. On the other hand, plant proteins, like grains, lack these essential amino acids. In addition to animal-based protein, veterinarians also recommend soy, dairy and eggs as protein sources.

Some animal proteins are high in copper, which is not good for liver disease. These should be avoided, especially organ meat like liver. Also avoid salmon, pork, lamb and duck since they are all rich in copper and go with chicken, turkey, beef and white fish instead.

Fats and Carbs

Again, depending on the case, some dogs with liver disease can tolerate higher levels of fat in their diet, while others should be kept at moderate fat intake. Fat is really important for energy and calories, but since it is processed through the liver, it can cause distress to dogs with liver disease. Therefore, it is best to feed only fats that are easily digestible, like coconut oil.

On the other hand, carbohydrates are important in all cases because they can help aid your dog's digestion since they are rich in fiber. They also help remove ammonia from your canine's system. Add white rice, oatmeal or pasta to your dog's diet.

Vitamin and Minerals

It is important to include vitamins like vitamin E, vitamin C, vitamin K, vitamin B complex and minerals like zinc. Vitamin C is good for its antioxidant properties, just like vitamin E, and they are great for liver health. They can lead to less inflammation in the liver, among other things.

Vitamin K can help with blood clotting and also assist your dog's body in coping with the byproducts of changed liver metabolism. Zinc is good for binding copper and also has antioxidant properties that help the liver function properly.

Structuring Your Dog's Liver Disease Diet

As we mentioned before, consult with your vet before you add any ingredients to your dog's diet and make sure to feed him at least four times a day.

Foods to Include

Eggs for dogs with liver disease. Add safe dairy products to your dog's diet, like ricotta cheese, cottage cheese and yogurt. These foods will help his digestion and will also produce less ammonia than meat. Just make sure that you stick to dairy products that are low in salt and fat and keep in mind that goat cheese is easier to digest than cow cheese.

Eggs are a great source of protein for your dog and you should include them in your diet. Other protein sources you can include are fish, and skinless and boneless turkey or chicken. These foods are high-quality proteins that are good for your dog's liver.

Oatmeal is great for liver disease because it contains soluble fiber that can help remove ammonia from your dog's system, which is good for the liver because it doesn't have to process it then. Boiled white rice is also something you should include in his diet because of soluble fiber, as well as barley and canned pumpkin.

Add a little bit of fish oil or salmon oil to your dog's meals because they are rich in omega-3 fatty acids and they can help reduce inflammation within the liver.

There is also a possibility that some fruits like watermelon, fig, and papaya can protect the liver, so try to include them in your dog's diet. However, if you want to feed your dog watermelon, then try to take out all the seeds because they can cause intestinal blockage. Also, don't give your dog more than a few figs because they can cause stomach upset.

Coconut, and especially coconut oil can be good for your dog's liver. Coconut oil is particularly good if your dog has trouble absorbing fat. Just add 1 tablespoon of coconut oil daily to your dog's diet, and use virgin or unrefined coconut oil.

Foods to Avoid

Avoid foods that are high in copper. Liver disease is associated sometimes with copper build-up and if that is the case with your dog, you should limit his copper intake. Most organ meats are high in copper, and you should particularly avoid beef liver. Chicken and turkey liver are fine since they have little copper. Avoid lamb, duck, pork and salmon as well.

Salt intake should be closely monitored because it can contribute to liver disease, particularly to retaining extra fluid. If your dog has a serious liver condition, you should put him on a low-salt diet. That will prevent the build-up of fluid in his abdomen.

Homemade Dog Food for Liver Disease

The best way to make sure that your dog isn't eating anything that can hurt his liver is to cook for him. There are many simple and easy recipes you can make quickly. Try the one I've mentioned below, and you can also try Samantha's liver disease recipe.

Homemade Diet for Dogs With Liver Shunt

What A Liver Shunt Is

A portosystemic shunt (PSS) or liver shunt is a disorder where the normal flow of blood, to and through the liver, is markedly reduced or even absent. Normally, blood returning from the puppy's digestive tract is routed to the liver through the portal vein. The blood flows through the liver and then exits the liver joining the venous blood flowing back to the heart. A liver shunt is a blood vessel that connects the portal vein with the main systemic blood stream. This causes the blood to bypass the liver.

When the puppy is just a fetus, the fetus' blood is carried from its body to the mother's and back again through the umbilical cord. The placenta is where the fetal blood and the mother's blood interact; although they never actually comingle. Nutrients from the mother's system are passed to the fetus and waste products from the fetus are taken up by the mother and processed through her kidneys and liver. The mother's liver then serves as the fetus' liver since the fetal liver is not yet capable of performing many important functions.

When the puppy is born, the umbilical cord is severed. Shortly after birth, the ductus venosus contracts, constricts, and closes. Once this vessel is closed off, the newborn pup's blood is forced to pass through the now developed liver. If the ductus venosus fails to close, then a portion of blood will continue to be shunted around the liver through the still patent ductus venosus.

How Much to Feed

The amount and how many times a day of food to feed daily depends on the breed of dog.

For pugs: one to eight years old is 1/2 to 3/4 cup of food twice daily.

There are many charts and feeding guidelines on the internet for each individual breed.

I serve Tess 1/4 cup of meat and top off the 1/2 cup measurement with a vegetable or veggie/ pasta mix that has been cooked. Some are mashed, some are boiled, and only a few are baked and considered a treat due to most vegetables having a higher sugar content when baked.

Tess' Activity & Family

Tess has survived the liver shunt for four years now. Every six months, she goes to see Doc Tom for her checkup and has passed every time. She shows no signs of slowing down or stopping. Tess loves to go swimming in any pond she can find, hiking many local trails, gardening, bounding through snow banks, and trips in the truck.

Tess lives with her birth sister, Gracie, has two cats, Finn & Poe, which she naps in the sun with and has fallen in love with Gilbert, who happens to be a mix of Black Lab and St. Bernard, and lives by the mailboxes she walks to daily.

Diet for Dogs With Canine Liver Disease

Following a dog liver disease diet is an important treatment tool for dogs with compromised liver function. A dietary change for a pet with canine liver disease (CLD) helps the liver regenerate while also maintaining good nutrition, so it's crucial to know what to feed a dog with liver problems.

Facts About Liver Disease in Dogs

Liver disease is common in dogs. It is especially prevalent in certain breeds such as West Highland Terriers and Doberman Pinschers. It is one of the top five causes of non-accidental canine deaths.

As the cleaning system for the body, the liver removes toxins and waste. It also produces bile for the digestive process. When the liver is compromised, toxins and waste may build up in the body. This may affect many of the other bodily systems such as the brain and heart.

The liver is remarkable in its ability to regenerate itself. With early detection and treatment, many CLD patients can recover completely.

Developing a Liver Diet for Dogs

While it's natural to wonder what's the best food to feed a dog with liver problems, please keep in mind that all significant diet changes should be thoroughly discussed with your veterinarian. CLD is not a condition that should be treated without medical guidance. Your vet will be able to structure a dietary plan that will help your pet recover.

As part of a treatment plan, a diet for dogs with liver disease includes four basic goals:

• Provide good nutrition to maintain energy and health

• Promote liver regeneration and reduce stress on the organ

• Prevent and minimize potential complications, such as hepatic encephalopathy, where the toxins affect the brain

• Preclude and inhibit liver damage from the accumulation of substances such as copper.

Specific Diet for Dogs With Liver Disease

Since dogs suffering from liver disease require a change in diet, there are specific steps to take with a dog's daily eating regimen. Of course, you will need to discuss your dog's specific needs with your veterinarian. Generally, your veterinarian will recommend a dog elevated liver enzymes diet based on commercially prepared or home-cooked meals, or a combination.

Prescription Liver Disease Diets

Prescription food for dogs with liver disease includes Hill's® Prescription Diet l®/d® and Royal Canin Veterinary Diet Canine Hepatic. Both of these low protein dog foods for liver disease come in wet and dry formulas. These diets are considered to be among the best options for dogs with liver diseases. If you decide on a prescription diet, follow the instructions on the package for your dog's weight. Break the meals up into about four or five smaller portions fed throughout the day rather than one big breakfast and dinner. This eases the stress on the body from processing a larger meal.

Dog Liver Detox Diet

A detox, or liver cleansing, diet, is made at home using fresh ingredients. Vet recommends a mixture of 25% white fish and 75% vegetables. Potential vegetables to consider adding include potatoes and sweet potatoes, green beans, squash, and zucchini. The site also recommends reducing the use of phenobarbital during the detox diet phase, but this should only be done in consultation with your veterinarian.

Additional Foods for Dogs With Liver Disease

Whether you are feeding prescription food or a home-cooked diet, add additional types of food to your dog's diet. Appropriate options include:

• Dairy products such as cottage cheese, yoghurt, goat cheese, and ricotta cheese.

• High-quality proteins such as chicken and turkey without the bones, fish, and eggs

• Oatmeal, white rice, barley and canned plain pumpkin (for soluble fiber)

• Fish oil (for the omega-3 fatty acids)

• Coconut oil

• Fruits such as blueberries, figs, seedless watermelon, and papayas

Protein Control

Your vet will most likely recommend a change in the protein consumption of your dog. Liver disease usually means that less protein is being processed, so your dog's protein intake will need to be monitored. The general recommendation is to ensure the protein consumed is high quality but to keep the amount to a moderate level. Some of the protein may come from non-meat sources such as cottage cheese. High-quality protein sources contain enough amino acids for your dog and are easily digested. Other recommendations may include offering plant-based proteins, such as soy, rather than meat-based proteins. In certain CLD complications, such as hepatic encephalopathy, the amount of protein may be reduced. Less protein will control the symptoms of that condition.

Copper Considerations

Some animal proteins contain high levels of copper and should be avoided in a liver disease diet for dogs. Organ meat, especially liver, should be avoided. Other meats high in copper include:

• Duck

• Lamb

• Salmon

• Pork

Protein sources that are relatively moderate to low in copper are:

• Turkey

• Chicken

• Whitefish

• Beef

• Eggs

• Cheese

• Fat

With CLD, dogs are able to tolerate higher levels of fat in the diet. Your vet may recommend a diet that has up to 50 percent fat content.

Carbohydrates

Carbohydrates are important to aid the digestion, add fiber and remove ammonia from the system. Cooked oatmeal, white rice, and pasta are types of carbohydrates that may be included.

Additives and Supplements

Dogs with CLD, especially in the advanced stages, should have a low-salt diet. Lowering salt prevents the build-up of fluid in the abdomen, called ascites which occurs in dogs with low liver function. There are good supplements that may help your dog with CLD. Some of these supplements are:

Vitamin B complex

Vitamin E

Zinc, which helps bind copper and has antioxidants which protect the liver

Vitamin C, for antioxidant action

Vitamin K, for blood clotting

Adenosylmethionine (SAMe), which may reduce liver injury and also has antioxidant properties

Commercial Diets

Your vet may prescribe a special commercial dog food. These prescription foods are specially designed for dogs with liver disease.

Feeding Routine

Some dogs with CLD benefit from a change in feeding routine. Instead of one or two regular meals a day, several small meals throughout the day may promote good digestion.

Getting Your Dog to Eat

Sometimes dogs with liver disease appear to lose their appetite. This could be because of the discomfort from the disease but also because the lower protein food may just be less palatable for them. If you need help getting a dog with liver disease to eat, trying one of the homemade diets might make a difference as this may be more enticing than dry kibble. If your vet agrees you can try mixing some of the prescription diet wet food with the kibble. You can also talk to your veterinarian about adding some fresh items to your dogs' food to increase their interest, such as a low sodium vegetable-broth or fresh veggies and fish.

Seek Veterinary Advice

If your dog has elevated liver enzymes, have a conversation with your vet about what that might mean in terms of your pet's health and diet. If your dog has liver disease, you should work with your vet to develop an appropriate canine liver disease diet for your pet. A good diet can help your dog feel better and heal faster.

WHY ISN'T MY OLDER DOG EATING

Dogs suffering from copper storage disease should not eat these recipes. Dogs diagnosed with Hepatic Encephalopathy may have problems with the protein in the following recipes.

CAN RAW BE THE ANSWER?

Many believe that feeding a raw diet can help dogs with liver disease. While this is the complete opposite of what you'll find here, I don't believe that it's not possible. I'm a huge fan of a raw diet and I recommend them all the time, however, this page is dedicated to feeding a home cooked diet for dogs diagnosed with Liver Disease.

These are the recipes that we've used for many of our own dogs when their liver enzymes weren't too extreme. You have to be very careful with this disease. This means that having your dog's blood work done routinely (every 6 months); including a complete liver profile is critical. If the liver enzymes remain stable, then you can continue with the diet; but, you have no way of knowing this information unless you have the blood work done on a regular basis.

The following homemade recipes for liver disease in dogs are for a week's worth of food and based upon our own dog's weight which was approximately 70-75 pounds at the time they were developed.

Also, you'll notice that there are no veggies included in the recipe and this is because our lab at the time had IBS and veggies can often cause soft stool and diarrhea.

Including desiccated liver in with the diet can also be a very good idea as a glandular therapy for dogs with liver disease and elevated liver enzymes.

RECIPES FOR DOGS WITH LIVER DISEASE

FISH & GROUND BEEF RECIPE FOR DOG WITH LIVER DISEASE

If your dog has elevated liver enzymes which could be due to ammonia in the blood (Hepatic Encephalopathy) or he or she is vomiting bile, this recipe is not ideal. Detoxing your dog first is the best thing to do for a dog with any type of liver issues PERIOD! This recipe can possibly be slowly incorporated later. See the link at the beginning of the page for immediate guidance.

D o NOT feed this recipe if your dog has copper storage disease. If you're not sure, ask your dog's vet if your has excessive amounts of copper in the liver. If you still don't know, treat your dog like he is storing copper and use the above link for immediate help.

Ingredients:

• 8 Cups of well-cooked brown rice (1560 grams)

• 7 Cups peeled, cooked and mashed sweet potato (1000 grams)

• 3 Cups cooked and chopped chicken livers (420 grams)

• 7 large hard-boiled eggs chopped

• 2 Cups poached, flaked, boneless haddock, cod or other whitefish (not tuna, shark or mackerel)

• 18 ounces regular ground beef, cooked in a little water but not overly browned

Preparation Method:

• Mix together and allow to cool completely. Stir in 1 tablespoon of fish oil.

- Next, YOU MUST and I repeat MUST add the following supplements in order to balance the diet:

- Calcium: Include 8-1/2 level teaspoons of pure calcium carbonate powder to the recipe.

- Iodine: Add 6 kelp tablets (take apart and sprinkle over the mixture).

- Zinc 50mg: Finely crushed and sprinkle THREE (3) through-out the food.

- Manganese 10mg Caps: Add TWO (2) finely crushed caps.

- Copper 2mg: Sprinkle SEVEN (7) of the capsule throughout the food.

- Coconut Oil: THIS SHOULD BE ADDED DAILY and NOT ALL ONCE -Add 1/2 teaspoon daily to your dog's food.

Using your hands, mix the food really good so that the supplements are mixed evenly through the food. Divide the food into 7 even batches and place in a freezer bag and freeze. Pull a bag out of the freezer the day before. Divide the bag into two meals for your dog that day.

CHICKEN AND SALMON RECIPE FOR DOGS WITH LIVER DISEASE

Again, if your dog has elevated liver enzymes which may be due to excess ammonia levels in the blood (Hepatic Encephalopathy) or he or she is vomiting bile, then detoxing your dog first is the best thing to do for any form of liver issues PERIOD! The recipe may be used later once your dog is stabilized.

Ingredients:

• 7 Cups well-cooked brown rice cooked very well (1365 grams)

• 2 Cups (measure out 2 cups of raw Quinoa) then cook (340 grams)

• 3 Cups peeled, cooked and mashed sweet potato (600 grams)

• 9 Cups lightly cooked ground chicken with fat (990 grams)

• 3 Ounces poached liver finely chopped

• 2 – 6 oz cans low sodium sockeye salmon (170grams per can)

Preparation Method:

• Allow this mixture to cool and stir in one tablespoon of fish oil. Add all of the following supplements.

• Calcium: Eight and one half (8.5) LEVEL teaspoons and sprinkle evenly over food. *Again, it should be notedthat Lulu was given 1 cup of cottage cheese daily effecting the amount needed in the recipe.

• Iodine: Sprinkle SIX (6) capsules evenly over the food.

• Zinc 50mg: Finely crush and sprinkle FOUR (4) evenly over food.

• Manganese 10mg: Finely crush and add ONE (1) evenly to food.

• NO COPPER NEEDED

• Coconut Oil: THIS SHOULD BE ADDED DAILY and NOT ALL AT ONCE -Add 1 teaspoon daily to your dog's food.

Using your hands, mix the food really good so that the supplements are mixed evenly through the food. Divide the food into 7 even daily portions and place them in individual freezer bags. Freeze and pull out what you need the day before. The bag is for two daily meals.

Carrot and Almond Butter Dog Treats (Recipe)

Golden, soft and chewy, these carrot and almond butter dog treats are sure to please your dog — and they look good enough for you to eat, too. Combine the wet ingredients in a bowl and mix well. Then, in a separate bowl, mix the dry ingredients.

Ingredients:

½ cup almond butter (all natural and organic, with no added sugar or salt)

¾ cup milk

1 egg

⅔ cup shredded carrot

1½ cups flour

1 tablespoon baking powder

⅓ cup oatmeal

Carrot and Almond Butter Dog Treats

Combine the wet and dry mixtures until a tacky dough forms.

Directions:

Heat your oven to 325 F.

In a medium bowl, combine the wet ingredients and mix well.

In a second bowl, stir together the flour, baking powder and oatmeal.

Combine the wet and dry mixtures until a tacky dough forms. If you use a stand mixer, you may have to switch to the dough hook.

Roll out the dough on a lightly floured surface to ¼-inch thickness and cut out shapes with a cookie cutter.

Place the biscuits on a nonstick baking sheet* and bake for 15 minutes.

Flip the biscuits over and bake for another 10 minutes.

If you don't have a nonstick baking sheet, you can line your baking sheet with parchment paper or a silicone baking mat.

This recipe makes about 2 dozen medium cookies.

If I know a treat is going to be soft and chewy, I often use a larger cookie cutter because I can hold the biscuit and let Banjo take bites without dry crumbs falling everywhere.

These carrot and almond butter dog treats cooked up to a perfect softness that made for an ideal large cookie.

Carrot Applesauce Dog Cookies (Recipe)

Got some leftover veggies? Try making these carrot applesauce dog cookies for a convenient — and healthy — treat for your pup. Carrots and flaxseed meal give these dog treats a nutrition boost. And when those ingredients happen to have added health benefits? Well, that's a win-win.

According to the American Kennel Club, "Carrots are an excellent source of vitamin A, potassium and fiber."

Ingredients:

½ cup rolled oats

½ cup unsweetened applesauce

½ cup shredded carrot

⅓ cup flour

¼ cup flaxseed meal*

*For pets with wheat allergies, coconut or almond flour would be a great substitute for the wheat flour. And if you don't have flaxseed meal on hand, you can increase the flour to ½ cup instead.

Bake for 20 minutes. This recipe makes about 1 dozen cookies.

Directions:

Heat your oven to 350 F.

In a medium bowl, combine all ingredients and mix well.

Drop the dough by tablespoons on a nonstick cookie sheet.

Bake for 20 minutes.

Banjo loved these carrot applesauce dog cookies, and I appreciated the chance to use up some leftover veggies.

Because this dog treat recipe is so simple, I had only a couple of dirty dishes afterward — which made cleanup a breeze.

Spinach, Apple and Carrot Dog Treats (Recipe)

This recipe gives you a great way to add a few fresh vegetables and fruit to your dog's diet — in the form of a delicious homemade treat.

Ingredients:

4 cups chickpea flour

1 teaspoon olive oil

2 eggs

½ cup baby carrots

1½ cups fresh spinach

½ apple, cored

¼ cup water

Puree the carrots, spinach, apple and water.

Directions:

Heat your oven to 350 F.

In a medium bowl, combine the flour, oil and eggs.

In a blender or food processor, puree the carrots, spinach, apple and water.

Stir the puree into the flour mix until it forms a sticky dough.

Drop tablespoon-sized dollops of the dough onto a nonstick baking sheet.

Bake for 15 minutes, until the treats are slightly browned along the edges and bottom.

This recipe makes about 3 dozen spinach, apple and carrot dog treats.

The color of these biscuits is a bright yellow with green speckling from all of the vegetables and chickpea flour. It's a nice change to the typical dirt-brown treats I'm used to.

Knowing that there are so many nutrients packed inside makes me really happy to feed them to Banjo.

Chickpea and Sardine Dog Treats (Recipe)

Sardine dog treats are a nutritious snack — those little fish have a lot of omega-3 fatty acids, yet they're also low in calories.

This sardine dog treats recipe requires just 3 ingredients: chickpea flour, sardines and eggs.

Ingredients:

2⅓ cups chickpea flour

3 tins of sardines (3.75 ounces each) packed in water, drained

2 eggs

Choose sardines packed in water rather than oil.

Directions:

Heat your oven to 350 F.

In a medium bowl, mix all ingredients.

Roll the dough out on a lightly floured surface to ¼-inch thick.

Cut out the biscuits and line them on a nonstick baking sheet.

Bake for 18–20 minutes for soft treats. Add a few minutes if you'd like them crispier.

Healthy Brewer's Yeast Dog Treats (Recipe)

Yes, brewer's yeast has health benefits for dogs, too. Here's how to make some irrestible brewer's yeast dog treats using this antioxidant-rich ingredient.

Did you know brewer's yeast is good for dogs? "brewer's yeast promotes healthy skin, hair, eyes and liver function" and "may reduce anxiety in dogs." Dr. Judith K. Herman DVM, CVH, agrees, saying, "Brewer's yeast is a great antioxidant."

Brewer's yeast is sometimes given as a supplement. But you can also use it as an ingredient in homemade dog treat recipes — like this one.

You can find brewer's yeast online or at your local health food store.

Ingredients:

2 cups rolled oats

1 cup brewer's yeast

1¼ cup flour

1 cup shredded cheddar cheese

1 egg, whisked

¾ cup water

Directions:

Heat your oven to 350 F.

In a large bowl, combine the oats, brewer's yeast, flour and cheese.

Mix in the whisked egg.

Add only as much of the water as necessary to create a rollable dough.

On a lightly floured surface, roll the dough out to ¼ inch.

Cut the dough with a cookie cutter and line the cookies on a nonstick sheet.

Bake for 20 minutes for soft treats and 30 minutes for crispier treats.

brewer's yeast dog biscuits

This recipe makes about 2 dozen brewer's yeast dog treats.

Vegan Banana Dog Treats (Recipe)

Ingredients:

2 tablespoons flaxseed meal

1 cup rolled oats

1 cup chickpea flour

1 teaspoon cinnamon

¼ teaspoon salt

1 banana, mashed

⅓ cup coconut oil, melted

If you use another type of flour (such as coconut flour or almond flour), you may need to add up to ¼ cup of water to reach a cookie dough consistency.

Bake them for 20 minutes. This recipe makes about 2 dozen vegan banana dog treats.

Directions:

Heat your oven to 350 F.

Combine the flaxseed meal, oats, flour, cinnamon and salt.

Mix in the mashed banana and coconut oil.

Drop the dough by tablespoons onto a non-stick cooking sheet and then flatten the balls with the back of a spoon.

Bake for 20 minutes.

Blueberry and Nut Butter Dog Treats (Recipe)

What's a gal to do when she has more blueberries than she can handle? Time to make some blueberry dog treats!

First, grind the oatmeal into a flour.

Ingredients:

1½ cups oatmeal

⅔ cup almond butter with no added salt or sugar

1 egg

¼ cup plain yogurt

¼ cup fresh blueberries

1 tablespoon honey

If the dough seems too runny, add a little more oatmeal.

Directions:

Using a food processor, grind the oatmeal until it resembles a coarse flour.

Add the remaining ingredients and process until smooth. If the dough seems too runny, add a little more oatmeal.

Press the dough between 2 sheets of wax paper and refrigerate for 20–30 minutes.

While you wait, heat your oven to 350 F.

Remove the dough from the fridge and, leaving it between the wax paper, roll it to ¼-inch thickness.

Using a knife or cookie cutter, cut out the treats and place them on a nonstick baking sheet.

Bake for 12–15 minutes.

This recipe makes about 2 dozen blueberry cookies for your dog.

Carob "Pupcakes" (Recipe for Healthy Dog-Friendly Cupcakes)

Ingredients:

Pupcakes:

2 tablespoons carob powder

½ cup flour

1 teaspoon baking powder

⅓ cup coconut oil, melted

⅓ cup plain Greek yogurt

1 egg

Coconut, sorghum, almond or rice flour would be preferable to a wheat flour.

Frosting (optional):

3 tablespoons plain Greek yogurt

1½ tablespoons almond butter or sunflower butter (organic, non-GMO)

There's enough batter in this recipe for 4 standard-size pupcakes or 12 mini pupcakes.

Directions:

Heat your oven to 350 F.

In a medium bowl, combine the dry ingredients.

In another medium bowl, whisk together the coconut oil, yogurt and egg.

Add the wet ingredients to the flour mixture and combine.

Scoop the pupcake batter into a nonstick or lined muffin pan.

Bake standard-size pupcakes for 20 minutes or mini pupcakes for 12 minutes.

While the pupcakes bake, mix together the frosting ingredients until well combined. Spoon the frosting into a sandwich bag and cut one corner off.

After the pupcakes have completely cooled, pipe the frosting on top.

Store any leftovers in the refrigerator.

After the pupcakes have completely cooled, pipe the frosting on top.

When I'm cooking for myself, I've found that carob is a lot like cocoa powder — it smells divine when it's baking, but if you don't add sugar to the recipe, the flavor is a little flat.

Beautiful Marbled Banana Carob Dog Cookies (Recipe)

This recipe takes a little longer to make because the final treats are a swirled combination of 2 separate doughs, creating a beautiful marbled effect.

Honey is a safe natural sweetener in small quantities.

Ingredients:

1 ripe banana

2 eggs

3 tablespoons honey

3 tablespoons olive oil

½ teaspoon cinnamon

½ teaspoon baking powder

2½ cups plus ¼ cup oat flour

¼ cup carob powder

Once you have these various light and dark balls, you pair them up (step 9 below).

Directions:

Heat your oven to 350 F.

Mash the banana with a fork in a medium bowl.

Mix in the eggs, oil, honey, cinnamon and baking powder.

Stir in 2½ cups flour.

Split the dough in half.

Add ¼ cup flour to one half of the dough and mix well.

Add ¼ cup carob powder to the other half of the dough and mix well. By now you should have one light dough ball without carob and one dark dough ball with carob.

Divide each half of the dough into 5 balls of dough.

Pair each smaller ball with one of the opposite color (i.e., one non-carob dough ball with one carob dough ball).

Roll each pair of dough balls out between 2 layers of plastic wrap to ¼-inch thick, and cut out with a cookie cutter.

Place cookies on a nonstick baking sheet and bake for 10 minutes. Flip them over and bake for another 10 minutes.

Use any cookie cutter you prefer.

Dried Banana Dog Chews (There's Just 1 Ingredient in This Recipe)

Ingredients:

Bananas (any amount)

Directions:

Heat your oven to 210 F.

Peel the bananas and slice them in half lengthwise, then cut each half in half lengthwise again.

Place the quartered bananas on a cooking sheet lined with parchment paper or a silicone baking mat.

Bake 2–4 hours, checking every half-hour. For shorter cooking time, create thinner slices.

The banana chews are done when they are dried and golden brown.

Grain-Free Black Bean Dog Cookies (Recipe)

The black beans make these treats look like chocolate cookies — except they're definitely dog-friendly.

Ingredients:

1 cup black beans, drained and rinsed well (from a 15 oz. can, low sodium)

¼ cup almond butter

½ very ripe banana

1 egg

Process until smooth, then refrigerate the batter for at least 1 hour.

Directions:

In a food processor, blend the beans until they create a paste.

Add the remaining ingredients and process until smooth.

Refrigerate the batter for at least 1 hour.

Heat your oven to 350 F.

Drop the dough by rounded teaspoons onto a nonstick cookie sheet.

Bake for 15 minutes.

Using the back of a fork, flatten the cookies.

Bake for another 10 minutes.

Flip the cookies over and bake for 20 more minutes.

Eggs And Chicken Mash

This meal certainly doesn't look appetizing. However, it can make your dog's day with a variety of flavors that it offers. The recipe uses quality protein sources that can be easily digested. It also includes fiber and carbs, making it a great mix of beneficial nutrients. This meal is really easy to make and is best served fresh.

Ingredients:

1 egg (boiled)

½ cup of oatmeal

¾ cup of cottage cheese (low fat)

½ cup of cooked chicken

½ cup of pumpkin (pureed or canned)

Preparation:

Cook, boil, or bake the chicken and then chop it into cubes.

Boil the egg and dice it into smaller pieces.

Take the oatmeal and cook it as well.

Now take all of the ingredients, add in pumpkin and mix them in a bowl.

Bring the meal to room temperature before you serve it.

Low Protein Veggie Cakes:

This recipe cuts back on protein and focuses more on green ingredients. You'll find a number of veggies in this recipe that provide carbs, fiber, and additional nourishment as well.

Ingredients:

1 cup of mixed vegetables (zucchini, squashes, sweet potatoes, starchy vegetables, etc.)

6 tablespoons of salt-free chicken broth.

2 and ½ cup of whole wheat flour.

1 and ½ cup of cold water

Preparation:

Bring your oven to 350 degrees Fahrenheit for preheating.

Cook all your vegetables and mash or puree them.

Add chicken broth to the veggie mix and then add flour.

Now steadily add cold water and mix until you form a dough.

Flatten out the dough and cut into smaller portion. Lay out these portions onto a baking tray.

Place the tray in the oven and bake the dough for 25 minutes.

Cool the cakes before you serve them or store them.

Doggy Pasta Salad

This is a rather simple meal that can be prepared at a moment's notice. It includes quality ingredients and is easy to digest. The amount of ingredients can be doubled if you have a bigger dog.

Ingredients:

½ package of any pasta.

2 eggs (hard boiled).

1 cup of brown rice.

½ packet of frozen broccoli.

Eggshell or bone meal for calcium (only if the vet approves it)

½ packet of frozen carrots.

Preparation:

Cook the pasta, brown rice, and vegetables.

Chop the eggs or mash them and then add them to a bowl.

Place the rest of your ingredients into the bowl and mix everything.

Bring the meal to room temperature and then serve it to your dog.

Molly's Massive Meatloaf Recipe.

INGREDIENTS:

- 5 lbs lean ground turkey

- 4 ounces of cheddar or other grated cheese

- 2 eggs

- 2 large mixing bowls

- 2 or 3 meatloaf cooking pans

- 1 1/2 carrots

- 1 1/2 sticks of celery

- 1 green pepper

- 1 lbs lean grown beef

- 1 apples or pears (take out the seeds)

- 1/2 cup string beans blanched

- 1/2 cup broccoli blanched

- 1/2 zucchini

- 1/2 sweet potato

- 1/2 cup of cooked brown rice

- Non-stick pan spray

DIRECTIONS:

1. Preheat the oven to 350F

2. Using a large bowl, mix the ground beef and turkey together, then place aside.

3. Grate up all your fruit and veggies with a food processor, then place them in a large bowl. If you do not have a food processor, you can use a cheese grater instead.

4. Add 2 eggs and 1/2 cup of cooked brown rice into the bowl full of grated veggies and fruit.

5. Place the grated veggies and fruit in with the ground meat and thoroughly mix all the ingredients together, before placing them into the meatloaf cooking trays. Remember to coat the trays with a non-stick spray before adding the meatloaf.

6. Place the meatloaf in the oven and cook on 350F for 90 minutes.

7. Once the meatloaf is finished cooking, drain off and discard any access liquid before letting the dish cool.

8.   Make sure that the meatloaf is completely cooled off before feeding it to your dog.

Maggie's Chicken Soup Recipe.

INGREDIENTS:

·   3 carrots

·   1 whole chicken or ½ a chicken depending on how much meat you want in the soup (you will have lots left over)

·   1 sweet potato

·   1 stock of celery

·   1 cup green beans

DIRECTIONS:

1. Place the chicken in a slow cooker with enough water to cover half of the chicken.

2. Turn the slow cooker on high heat and cook for 6 hours

3. Dice up all the veggies and place them in a pot with 1 cup of water.

4. Place the pot on the stove and allow to simmer for 1 hour.

5. Once the chicken has finished cooking, remove it from the slow cooker and allow to cool.

6. One the chicken has Cooled, remove and discard the skin.

7. Skim and discard the fat from the broth which is left behind in the crockpot.

8. Add 1/2 cup of the broth to the simmering pot of veggies.

9. Shred up the desired amount chicken and add it to the pot of veggies.

10.   Stir the mix thoroughly, then allow to fully cool before serving to your dog.

Buddy's Beef And Veggie Crockpot Recipe.

INGREDIENTS:

- 2 1/2 lbs ground beef

- 2 tbsp of olive oil

- 1 1/2 cups chopped butternut squash

- 1 1/2 cups cooked brown rice

- 1 1/2 cups chopped carrots

- 1 (15-ounce) can kidney beans, drained and rinsed

- 1/2 cup peas, frozen or canned

DIRECTIONS:

1. Add the cooked brown rice, kidney beans, butternut squash, carrots and ground beef into a slow cooker with 4 cups water.

2. Cook on low heat for 8-9 hours, then add the frozen peas before cooking for another 30 minutes.

3. When finished, drain off the excess liquid, then add 2 tbsp of olive oil before stirring the mix into a mash or using a food processor.

4. Let the mix cool completely before serving it to your dog.

Max's Turkey & Liver Mash Recipe.

INGREDIENTS:

- 2 lbs lean ground turkey.

- 1/2 lb raw beef liver.

- 2 Carrots.

- 2 tablespoons olive oil.

- 1 cups of cauliflower.

- 1 cup of broccoli florets.

- 1 cup of zucchini.

DIRECTIONS:

1. Place all the vegetables in a steamer or boil them until tender, about 10 to 20 minutes.

2. After the vegetables are finished being steamed and allowed to cool, place them into a food processor or cut them up by hand. The chopping size will depend on the consistency you would like to obtain.

3. Fry or boil the liver on medium-high heat until cooked through. If frying, keep all the access fats which are high in nutrients and can be added to the mix.

4. Place all the cooked ingredients into a large mixing bowl before adding 2 tbsp of olive oil and stirring the mix into a mash by hand or food processor.

5. Let the mix cool completely before feeding it to your pet.

Charlie's Turkey Meatball Treats Recipe.

INGREDIENTS:

·	1 lbs of lean ground turkey

·	1 cup of breadcrumbs

·	1 cup of raw chopped cranberries. (Make sure to remove the pits)

·	1 cup of green beans

DIRECTIONS:

1. Preheat oven to 350°F before adding all your ingredients into a large mixing bowl.

2. Thoroughly mix everything together by hand or food processor before rolling the meatballs into shape with your hands.

3. Place the meatballs in the oven and let them cook for 40 to 60 minutes.

4. Make sure to let the meatballs cool off completely before feeding them to your dog.

Molly's Massive Meatloaf Recipe.

INGREDIENTS:

- 5 lbs lean ground turkey

- 4 ounces of cheddar or other grated cheese

- 2 eggs

- 2 large mixing bowls

- 2 or 3 meatloaf cooking pans

- 1 1/2 carrots

- 1 1/2 sticks of celery

- 1 green pepper

- 1 lbs lean grown beef

- 1 apples or pears (take out the seeds)

- 1/2 cup string beans blanched

- 1/2 cup broccoli blanched

- 1/2 zucchini

- 1/2 sweet potato

- 1/2 cup of cooked brown rice

- Non-stick pan spray

DIRECTIONS:

1. Preheat the oven to 350F

2. Using a large bowl, mix the ground beef and turkey together, then place aside.

3. Grate up all your fruit and veggies with a food processor, then place them in a large bowl. If you do not have a food processor, you can use a cheese grater instead.

4. Add 2 eggs and 1/2 cup of cooked brown rice into the bowl full of grated veggies and fruit.

5. Place the grated veggies and fruit in with the ground meat and thoroughly mix all the ingredients together, before placing them into the meatloaf cooking trays. Remember to coat the trays with a non-stick spray before adding the meatloaf.

6. Place the meatloaf in the oven and cook on 350F for 90 minutes.

7. Once the meatloaf is finished cooking, drain off and discard any access liquid before letting the dish cool.

8. Make sure that the meatloaf is completely cooled off before feeding it to your dog.

Liver Boosting Meal

This recipe makes use of ingredients that boost the liver's functioning and regeneration. You can also add various supplements to it to make it even more beneficial. Keep in mind that supplements should only be given if your vet prescribes them. Even without any supplements, this recipe can fill your dog's belly with superb nutrients.

Ingredients:

1 Lb. of boneless chicken thighs.

1 red bell pepper.

5 cups of water.

2 cups of white rice.

1 Brazil nut.

2 and ½ teaspoons of eggshell (crushed or powdered).

3 tablespoons of sunflower seed oil.

2 cups of cottage cheese (low fat).

Preparation:

Dice chicken into tiny cubes (about ½ inch cubes).

Slice bell pepper and remove any seeds from it.

Add the bell pepper, chicken, and rice to 5 cups of boiling water. Let the mixture cook at low heat until water is almost completely reduced.

Take eggshell, sunflower seed oil, and any supplements that you've been prescribed and blend them into a fine mixture.

Add the blended mixture into the cooked rice, bell pepper, and chicken mixture. Add cheese and mix well.

Serve the mixture while it's lukewarm. You can also store it for up to 5 days.

These dog food recipes are easy to make and are designed to carry as many useful nutrients as possible. They only make use of easily digestible ingredients, making sure that your dog's meals don't stress out their liver. A proper diet is essential when it comes to fighting CLD. It gives your dog's body the relief and nourishment needed to heal. Also, while a proper diet is necessary, you shouldn't forget about proper medication.

A proper diet will help your dog's liver heal and de-stress. Proper and timely medication will keep the disease from worsening. Make sure that you regularly visit your vet and follow whatever guidelines that they give you. With the right care, your dog will continue to have a comfortable and joyful life.

Cooked Chicken with Cottage Cheese

This homemade dog food recipe is good for dogs with liver disease because it has high-quality protein in chicken, cheese and egg, but it is also rich with soluble fiber from oatmeal and pumpkin, which will help his digestion as well. It is also a pretty simple recipe that requires only around 20 minutes of prep time.

Ingredients:

3/4 cup of low-fat cottage cheese

1/2 cup of cooked chicken

1/2 cup of cooked oatmeal

1 boiled egg

1/2 cup of canned pumpkin

Preparation:

The Guide on How to Feed Dogs With Liver Disease. The first thing to do is to cook the chicken. You can use chicken breasts if you want to stick to lean, low-fat meat, but other parts of chicken meat are also fine. Just make sure that it is boneless and skinless. Dice the chicken meat and then bake it, cook it in a frying pan or boil it, whatever you prefer.

Cook the oatmeal and boil the egg in advance and when your chicken is thoroughly cooked, just mix these ingredients together. After that, add cottage cheese and canned pumpkin and mix it all in one large bowl.

As soon as you mix it properly, you can serve this meal to your dog. You can store leftovers in your fridge for up to 4 days, and if you make a larger batch you can also freeze it for up to 2 months.

Homemade Dog Food for Liver Disease

If you are making your own food, feed at least 50% of the meals as meat, keeping carbs and grains under 50% or less. You can calculate the amount of food for your dog by multiplying one gram of protein times your dog's body weight.

I recommend a liver cleansing diet, which consists of a 50/50 mix of white potatoes and sweet potatoes with a white fish such as cod and halibut.

Mix 1/3 fish to 2/3 potato mixture. As the dog acclimates to the diet, you can add cooked chopped carrots, yellow squash and green beans, and scrambled eggs.

CONCLUSION

Dietary changes of any kind should be made slowly. Doing it fast can hurt your dog's stomach and make him feel worse than before. Talk with your vet to determine how to incorporate these changes.

Try to feed your dog several times every day, not just one or two meals. Stick to smaller meals and feed him 4-5 times a day to make it easier on his stomach and decrease the amount of nutrition the liver has to process.

Some holistic vets may recommend to avoid commercial dog food brands altogether since they often contain proteins, grains and starches that may negatively affect the liver. There is no clear evidence to prove one way or another at the moment, but certain dog food brands may be better than others. If, however, you choose to feed your dog a homemade dog food diet for liver disease, this article will explain dietary guidelines for it.